Mastery of Nourishing Bone Broth: Unveiling Secrets for Healthiness : The Ultimate Guide to Boosting Immunity and Rejuvenating Your Body with Bone Broth.

*<u>**Funny helpful tips:**</u>*

Invest in digital marketing; online visibility drives sales in today's market.

Engage with books that promote creativity; they stimulate the imagination and innovative thinking.

Life advices:

Your journey is a testament to your resilience; honor each step, knowing it has shaped you.

Cultivate a diverse network; varied perspectives enrich your understanding and approach.

Introduction

This book serves as a comprehensive guide to harnessing the health benefits and culinary versatility of bone broth. It starts with a brief overview of cooking bone broths, including differentiating between broth, bone broth, stock, and commercially available products. The guide delves into essential topics such as choosing bones, preserving them, and easy cooking methods for preparing bone broth at home.

Readers will learn how to discern high-quality bone broth and the best practices for storing it to maintain its freshness and nutritional integrity. The cookbook then introduces the 21-day bone broth diet plan, providing a structured approach to incorporating bone broth into a balanced diet for health and wellness.

The recipes section features basic bone broths, including classic chicken, duck, turkey, pork, beef, lamb, fish, and venison variations. Each recipe is meticulously crafted to extract maximum flavor and nutrients from the bones, offering a foundation for creating nourishing soups, stews, and main dishes.

For those seeking specialized health benefits, the cookbook presents health-boosting bone broths tailored to enhance skin health, immunity, energy, and gut function. These recipes are designed to address specific wellness goals and support overall health and vitality.

In addition to traditional soups and stews, the cookbook provides innovative recipes for incorporating bone broth into main dishes, such as spring vegetable soup, beefy vegetable soup, and curried lentil soup with coconut milk. Readers will also discover recipes for homemade bouillon and sauces, showcasing the versatility of bone broth in enhancing flavor and nutrition in everyday cooking.

The cookbook doesn't stop at culinary applications; it also explores bone broth remedies for common health concerns, including allergies, coughs, weight management, fever relief, and detoxification. With easy-to-follow recipes and practical tips, readers can harness the healing power of bone broth to support overall well-being.

For those wondering where to source bones for making bone broth, the cookbook offers guidance on finding quality bones, including feet, knuckles, and other sources at whole food markets, online, and specialty stores. It also provides insights into enhancing bone broth with additional ingredients and highlights other health benefits beyond its nutritional profile, such as detoxification, digestion, joint support, immune system function, and improved sleep quality.

In essence, this book serves as a comprehensive resource for anyone looking to incorporate nutrient-rich bone broth into their daily diet for improved health and vitality.

Contents

CHAPTER 1

A BRIEF GUIDE TO COOKING BONE BROTHS

Contrary to what many people think, the bone broth diet is not just a trend that will soon fade away. Broths have been a daily part of the human diet for hundreds of years, so much so that they are often turned to as a treatment to many ailments, from stomach pain and coughs to inflammation and lethargy even up to this day.

Our early hunter-gatherer ancestors made bone broth mainly because it was essential to their survival; essential that they used every part of each animal they killed or caught as hunting was a difficult and dangerous part of life. They mastered the use of all the parts of every animal and ate as much as possible then used the bits they could not eat to make tools, weapons, clothing and shelters.

Our early ancestors learned that heat would help to break down the tough parts of animals and release the nutrients they contained. As far back as 20,000 years ago, during the last great Ice Age in China people were cooking their food in pots according to the evidence found, the remains of small, crude, fired clay pots found while excavating in Xianrendong Cave Southeast China.

The first evidence of early pottery found, a small statue of a naked woman that was dated from about 300,000 years ago was found in the Czech Republic. It is probable that these early humans also started moulding clay into pots and jars for storage soon after this time.

Making broth in crude pots does not sound so exciting or important but it was the beginning of modern cooking. Once a broth was made other things such as tubers, vegetables that could not be eaten raw, seeds and grains, herbs and spices could have been added to make full meals. This development made life suddenly much easier especially for our early ancestors who live in these harsh and cold areas.

By 12,000 BC the art of cooking was well established in many of the regions of the world. In Asia bone broth became a staple part of many different cuisines, a variety of Chinese meals feature a bone broth type soup to help cleanse the palate and aid with digestion. In Korea Seolleongtang a bone broth is made using Ox brisket and bones. Japanese Tonkotsu, a noodle soup, is made using broth made from pork bones.

In Ancient Greece Hippocrates the Father of Modern Medicine was known to recommend bone broth to patients with digestive issues.

Maimonides, a Middle Eastern Philosopher and Physician recommended the use of chicken bone broth as a remedy for many conditions such as colds flu, a healthy preventative measure as well as being a tasty meal. His recommendation seems to have stood the test of time with many people swearing on the benefits of chicken soup. It is even known by many as the "Jewish Penicillin" because of its therapeutic effects.

Bone broth was and still is widely used in South America and even spread to the Caribbean where it is often used as part of many types of common healthy breakfasts.

Bone broth is indeed more than just your grandmother's favorite all-around remedy, because it does contain the nutrients needed to help the body maintain healthy organs and repair damaged cells. It is rich in calcium, magnesium, potassium, and phosphorus as well as the amino acids proline and glycine, all of which help maintain healthy bones, joints, cartilage, internal organs, and even hair, skin, and nails. Collagen, an important protein that is naturally found in the body and gives the skin its natural elasticity, can be supplemented by bone broth as well.

With the beginning of the industrial revolution, new forms of technology saw an increase of the usage of bone broth. Gelatine from broth became very popular to make healthy desserts as well as being used in fine dining for sauces, gravies, soups stews and confectionary.

Because it is time consuming to make and can use a lot of energy to produce it at home, bone broth soon became a massed produced product that people purchased in cans, dried in powder form or dried cubes for to make their own instant broth at home.

While being very convenient almost all the vital and important nutrients in the bone broth are lost during processing and the flavor is also reduced.

About this time, approximately 1908 artificial Monosodium Glutamate (MSG) was invented by a Japanese biochemist; its main purpose was to emulate meat flavoring.

Unfortunately, many large food manufacturers and processors adopted or started using MSG to make their product taste like they had meat in them and save on a huge amount of food costs. Now, most of the commercial bone broth or stock you can buy is not even made using bones, some of the better commercial Bone broths, while they are made using bones, the bones and other ingredients come from factory farmed livestock. These products are best avoided as they contain many chemicals and additives that are often given to factory farmed livestock.

Fortunately, there is a large resurgence in the use of homemade bone broth; it has become one of the most common health foods people consume with many discerning consumers refusing the mass-produced commercially available chemically laden types. Healthy homemade bone broths made with the best organic ingredients such as your grand and great grandparent as well as all the generations before them, enjoyed and grew up with.

WHAT IS THE DIFFERENCE BETWEEN BROTH, BONE BROTH, STOCK, THE HOMEMADE VERSIONS AND THE COMMERCIALLY AVAILABLE PRODUCTS?

Many people use these terms interchangeably and do not really distinguish between them, Broth, Bone Broth and Stock all are very similar, but they have several unique differences

- Broth is normally or typically made using meat and possibly a small amount of bone cooked in water. When you boil or poach a chicken, the liquid that is left over when the chicken is removed is a basic broth. Often there are vegetables, herbs and spices added to enrich the taste of the chicken and subsequently the broth. Usually depending on the age of the bird or type of meat you are cooking the cooking time is relatively short, just enough to cook and tenderize the meat. For chicken or other poultry between 45 minutes and 3 hours. For red meats such as pickled pork or corned beef anywhere from 1 hour to 4 hours is the usual cooking time. The normal broth is very light in flavor and often thin in

4

texture, but does often contain a lot of protein as well as fats. It is usually used for the base of a soup, stew or other dishes that require liquids.

- Stock is normally or typically made using bones with some meat still attached; it often includes tendons sinew and gristle. An acid such as vinegar or citrus juice is also added to help the release of minerals from the bones. Usually but not always vegetables such as root crops, carrots, parsnips, swedes and onions, garlic, celery are added to boost flavor and the nutritional content. Aromatics such as selected herbs and spices, pepper, ginger, chili, cumin, fenugreek, cardamom, basil, sage, rosemary, thyme bay leaves, star anise and many more are added to obtain the desired flavor.

- .Some stocks are made for special dishes, while others are made to be used in more general applications. It is usual to roast the bones and the vegetable before making the stock to bring out the flavors and give richness and body to the stock. Another reason for roasting is it takes away the tendency of stocks to taste slightly bitter. Stocks are usually cooked within moderately short times, depending on the type of bones being used. Fish, 30 minutes to 2 hours, Poultry, 3 to 4 hours, Red Meats 4 to 12 hours. Stocks are very healthy and contain large amounts of gelatin, so are high in protein and also contain many trace nutrients.

- Bone Broth is usually or typically made using only bones, but can contain a small amount of meat that has adhered to the bone. Most people blanch the bones first to remove any impurities and then roast them in the same way as mentioned when making stock, as this will greatly improve the color and flavor of the broth. An acid such as vinegar or citrus juice is also added to help leach out the minerals and other nutrients from the bones. Unlike simple broth and stocks, bone broths require very long cooking times or more correctly simmering times.

Fish and other seafood are from 3 to 12 hours, Poultry 5 to 18 hours, Red Meats 12 to 72 hours. The purpose in the long cooking times is to produce gelatin which comes from their collagen content but also to obtain from the bones their essential trace mineral content. Sometimes at the end of the cooking time the bones are reduced to the stage they easily crumble. If they remain strong they can be used again; many large thick bones can be used many times before their full wealth of nutrients are recovered.

Bone broths are extremely rich in protein as well as a good source of trace minerals. It is a good source of Glycine which helps with digestion, the secretion of gastric acid, making bile salts and supports our body's detoxification processes as well as being used during the synthesis of hemoglobin. It is also high in Proline which helps with good skin health and the high gelatin content is especially helpful in healing stomach and intestine disorders.

HOW TO CHOOSE THE BONES

The thing about bone broths is that you should not just use any bones you may find in the market. In fact, it is crucial for you to choose the best quality, organic bones. Of course, this is not just to make some fancy broth, because in order for you to get the best possible nutrients, you need well-fed and well cared for animal meat and bones. These should be guaranteed grass-fed beef, sheep, veal, bison or buffalo, pasture-raised and organic-fed chicken, duck, turkey, and pork bones.

When it comes to choosing the best parts in organic, grass-fed beef, it is advised that you get the knuckle-bones, oxtail, feet, and beef shank as these have the highest amount of gelatin. In pork, choose the feet and knuckle-bones. Poultry heads and feet are also rich in gelatin and nutrients, even though it may seem a little off-putting to some people. Do not worry for you will be discarding the solids at the end of cooking time, so you will only be left with the nutrients in the broth.

It's always good to have some variety when making use of bone broth. For one, you can use red marrow, which can be found in the skull, sternum, hip bone, scapula, vertebra, ribs, and the long end of beef or chicken's bones. Red marrow could be quite amazing because it's where you can find the stem cells, and stem cells can help build up your immune function and strength—and you will easily get that once you use this kind of broth.

On the other hand, you can also use yellow marrow—the most common kind—which is found in the central portion of the bone, and where fats are stored.

If you're still confused, it would be best to just keep in mind that aside from beef, and chicken, you can use an assortment of animals, but it would be best to make sure that those animals are free-range, pastured, or grass-fed, and that they're fed with organic produce so that you can be sure that it's clean, and that it has all the nutrients you need.

If you're going to be using large bones, do go ahead and cut them up into small pieces, if you can. Doing so would make way for better boiling and easier absorption of the minerals. It also allows more material to be used as part of the broth.

You can buy the bones for your broth from a guaranteed organic local farm, a local butcher whom you trust would provide you the 100 percent organic kind, or at a meat department of a reputed local health food store. Some can even order their organic bones from reliable online sources. If you think high quality bones are a little too costly, you would be happy to know that you can reuse the bones for multiple broth batches until they start to become too soft. In this sense, it is money well-spent.

You can also use leftover bones from an already cooked animal for your bone broth. Whatever bones are left on the serving dish after all the guests have consumed, the turkey can be used, as well as any leftover bones from a roasted pig.

Seafood broth can be made from the shells of any mollusk or crustaceans as well as the bones heads scales and other trimmings of fresh fish. The main difference is if using shells and crustaceans such as shrimp, prawn, crab, lobster or crayfish the water should only be allowed to simmer gently for 30 minutes then the shells should be strained from the broth as after this time the broth can become bitter. During the simmering time gently remove any foam that appears on the surface and discard this as it will hold any impurities from the shells. This broth can be used as is or added to a fish bone broth to further enhance both.

HOW TO PRESERVE THE BONES

The best type of bones for high quality bone broth should be the newly roasted ones or freshly bought ones from your local farmer or butcher. Once you have got the bones in your kitchen, you should immediately wrap them up in wax paper or plastic and freeze them. Each time you plan on re-using the bones for making bone broth, simply unwrap them and plunk them into a stock pot along with measured out water, vinegar, and salt.

If like us you make a lot of fresh broth and therefore use lots of bones it can become difficult to find enough space in which to store the bones. After they have been used once, it is possible and often preferable to dry the bones and hang them if you have a good place to do this. They must be hung in a cool, dry area out of direct sunlight

First, wash the bones to be reused to ensure there are no extra pieces with them and then dry the bones through in the oven on a medium temperature. Once completely dry lightly wrap them in brown paper to stop any dust or airborne contaminants reaching them, and hang them until needed. A great place to hang them we find is in our garage just under the roof, it is well ventilated and safe from pests the weather and easy to access.

EASY BONE BROTH COOKING METHODS

Nowadays, not everyone has the luxury of keeping an eye on a bubbling stock pot over a stovetop for 72 hours. Fortunately, you do not necessarily have to do that if two other options are available to you: pressure cooking and slow cooking (or using a Crockpot).

When you use a pressure cooker, you will only have to watch your stovetop for 3 hours, while slow cookers can do the job on their own for several hours (24 to 48 hours, on average) without you checking up on it so often. If you still decide to choose the stovetop, never leave your boiling broth alone because you certainly would not want to end up losing your home to a fire just for the sake of some bone broth, no matter how delicious it is.

The ratio for cooking bone broth is pretty simple: 1 pound (or 0.45 kg) of bones to 1 quart (or 0.9 liter) water, along with 1/2 tablespoon of acid (citrus or vinegar) and 1 teaspoon of salt per pound of bones.

Whatever method you use, you must remember to include an acid, such as citrus (lemon or lime juice) or a mild vinegar (such as rice wine or apple cider vinegar). The acid will draw out the minerals from the bones easily and transfer it to the broth.

You might notice that the basic bone broth recipes in this cookbook do not call for an addition of vegetables such as onions, garlic, carrots, celery, and so on. This is because vegetables will break down more quickly compared with bones, and at the end of cooking time, the precious nutrients from these would have already dissipated. However, if you do want to add them, you must only stir them in near the end of cooking time if not right after.

HOW TO TELL IF IT IS HIGH QUALITY BONE BROTH

The easiest way to tell if your bone broth is chock full of nutrients you want in it is by putting it in the refrigerator and then checking to see if it becomes gelatinous once cooled.

If your broth did not end up like that, then what you can do add more bones. Non-organic bones are also less likely to give you this type of result, so make sure to only use organic and cruelty-free ones (because it means the animals were well-fed and given enough nutrients and exercise to promote proper nutrient absorption).

Other tips are to use a bit more vinegar or lemon juice and ensure that the broth goes to boiling point during cooking time. It would also help to give it even more time to cook.

HOW TO STORE BONE BROTH

Once you have your finished product, you need to separate the solids from your broth. Use a mesh sieve to do this. If the bones are still a good candidate for re-use, then let them cool and then wrap them up and store them in the freezer. If they become quite tender, you may choose to grind them in a high power food processor or blender so that any remaining goodness in them can be given to your pets.

The best container to store bone broths in the refrigerator would be glass ones, such as mason jars. If the lids of your glass jars become rusty, then simply buy plastic lids as replacement.

If you want to freeze the broth in a glass jar, make sure that there is 2 inches or more of head-space between the lid and the surface of the broth, otherwise the glass jar will break once the broth freezes over and expands. Some bone broth fanatics love to pour their bone broths in ice trays instead, so that whenever they need some all they have to do is pop the cubes into a pan and reheat on the stovetop.

Different sized ice cube trays are readily available so you can have a range of broth in convenient ready to use sizes. This makes having a cup or two of amazing healthy bone broth as easy as making instant coffee or teabag tea. Just place a frozen cube or two of broth in a cup and add boiling water, a sprinkling of fresh parsley or your favorite herb and maybe a little natural unrefined sea or rock salt

If you do not have freezer space, a good method is to reduce the broth to a concentrate. This can be done using a crock-pot or another alternative is using shallow baking dishes in the oven on the lowest setting. This is probably the quickest method. Place the broth to about 1.5in deep in the oven dishes and reduce it in the oven, over a few hours.

Another tried and true method is to make Portable Broth or Soup, this method has been used for thousands of years by travelers and adventures. There is a good recipe for making this in the chapter on soups later in this book.

Once the broth is reduced to a thick and very gelatinous type of syrup, it can be further dried to form usually into a solid nugget or flat biscuit so it could easily be carried in a pocket and then when needed easily and quickly reconstituted to a delicious, healthy soup or base for a stew.

If you are fortunate enough to have a dehydrator you can make your own homemade bone broth powder. Once the broth is reduced to a very thick syrup type consistency it can be spread onto the drying trays or mats and allowed to dehydrate until it loses all its moisture. It then forms into a very brittle, glass-like sheet. This sheet can easily be broken into pieces and then placed in a food processor or blend. It then only takes a few seconds to form a fine dry powder. This bone broth powder can be stored in a food safe, airtight container at room temperature until required. It makes an excellent food flavor booster and can be used in place of broth/stock or even just sprinkled on food such as cheese on toast or egg dishes.

THE BEST BONE BROTH COOKING PRACTICES TO ENSURE HEALTHY DELICIOUS BROTH

Bone broth is now making a comeback to where it was several generations ago because of its incredible health properties as a mainstay in most kitchens whether you use it as a miracle cure for almost all your ailments or just as a hearty hot drink to warm you up over the colder months of the year. When you make a bone broth it is worth making the best broth possible.

A poorly made bone broth is about as palatable as chewing on an old dry bone.

1. The first step when starting is to blanch the bones, this is done to remove any extras or impurities that may come with the bones. Usually when using the best natural bones for making bone broth such as feet, knuckles, marrow necks and heads, the parts with large amounts of collagen. These bones can also contain a few extras that you do not want so blanching is the best option.

The collagen causes the broth to become gelatinous at normal room temperatures. If this happens it shows that you have done it right and made a great brew. If your broth is thin and watery at room temperature or when refrigerated then it is either made with bones from feedlot livestock that do not contain the correct nutrients that they should contain, if they were from natural pasture fed organic livestock or you just need more bones and less water.

To blanch the bones, cover them with pure fresh water and bring them to the boil for about 20 minutes then drain and roast.

2. Roasting the Bones; One of the joys of bone broth is the rich flavors you get when it's made properly. Always roast the bones when you make bone broth to get the rich and satisfying flavors and colors. Most bones will need to be roasted for about 45 minutes, not burnt, but caramelized and browned. After roasting it is worthwhile to include all the drippings at the bottom of your pan. Just scrape them into the pot to help give some extra depth of flavour to the finished broth.

3. Many people like to add a variety of different stuff to the bone broth in an effort to try and improve the quality, nutritional value and flavour; don't add anything except an acid such as vinegar or lemon juice. Because of the long cooking times all nutrients in anything apart from the bones will be lost. The vinegar (acid helps to release the minerals and other locked in nutrients from the bones.

Bones tendons, cartilage and marrow contain nutrients such as amino acids, glucosamine and chondroitin, Minerals including boron, magnesium, phosphorus, silicon and sulphur, as well as other trace minerals, these are all in forms that are readily absorbed by our body's, unlike many supplements.

If you want to add aromatics to your bone broth, that should be done during the last 30 minutes to 1 hour of cooking time. Or better yet, finish the broth and take the amount of broth want to consume and place your additions such as fresh or roasted vegetables, herbs spices and other aromatics into this in a separate saucepan

4. It is important to use a large enough pot to take the bone you're using and place in it enough water to just cover them, not to drown them, some bones are very large and these can be cut with a bone saw or broken with a hammer before cooking.

5. Make sure you simmer your bone broth for the right length of time at least 12 hours and up to 72 hours for red meat bones and 6 to 12 hours for fine bones like chicken or small birds.

6. Cooling and storing your Bone Broth. Work out the best method to cool down your finished bone broth as soon as possible after you finish cooking it. This is important as hot can be a breeding ground for bacteria. The danger zone for all food is between 40F (4.4C) and 140F (60C). Food between these temperatures is a breeding ground for bad and dangerous bacteria. If you have a large amount of bone broth in a stockpot a good method to cool it quickly is to place the pot in a larger bowl of icy water, and keep adding ice to reduce the temperature quickly. Stirring will also help bring the hot liquid to the cold outside. It is also reasonable to put a few cups of clean ice inside with the broth as this will not noticeably dilute the broth.

Do not place hot broth directly into the refrigerator as this will raise the temperature inside the refrigerator and possibly lead to bacteria multiplying rapidly and the contamination of other items there. It is best to freeze the bone broth within 2 hours of being made.

See, cooking broths do not seem so difficult now. The process is straight forward and minimal enough, so get to cooking!

CHAPTER 2

THE 21-DAY BONE BROTH DIET PLAN

The following diet plan does not have to be followed strictly; it is simply meant as a guide that you can print out and then stick on the refrigerator door to help get you into the bone broth habit.

Feel free to make some changes to the ingredients depending on whatever products are available in your area. For instance, you can choose any other cruciferous vegetable for the **Cream of Cauliflower Soup** if you are not a big fan of cauliflowers. What matters is that you are able to sneak in some bone broth into your diet every day.

Also, do keep in mind that the meals mentioned here are made with bone broth—and when you eat them for at least 3 weeks, you'd definitely notice positive things happening for your health—and your life. You can make variations of them, and do whatever you want—as long as bone broth is in the mix, or is part of any of your meals for the day.

DAY 1:

Breakfast: Artichoke Curried Scramble with sun-dried tomatoes

Lunch: Classic Chicken Bone Broth

Snacks: Lime and Coconut Sipping Broth

Dinner: Spiced Cranberry Pot Roast

DAY 2:

Breakfast: Cream of Cauliflower Soup

Lunch: Ginger, Beet, and Coconut Soup

Snacks: Stuffed Cabbage

Dinner: Shrimp Gumbo

DAY 3:

Breakfast: Shepherd's Pie

Lunch: Slow Cooker Caveman Chili

Snacks: Fish Bone Broth

Dinner: Beef Shanks with Vietnamese Spiced Glaze

DAY 4:

Breakfast: Apple Maple Chicken Breakfast Sausage

Lunch: Spring Vegetable Soup

Snacks: Sloppy Lettuce Wraps

Dinner: Bacon-wrapped Filet Mignon with Paleo Pan Sauce

DAY 5:

Breakfast: Classic Beef Bone Broth

Lunch: Chicken Broccoli Casserole

Snacks: Ginger Leek Beef Sipping Broth

Dinner: Broth Burgers

DAY 6:

Breakfast: Beefy Vegetable Soup

Lunch: Pork Chops with Pear Shallot Sauce

Snacks: Osso Busco with sun-dried tomatoes

Dinner: Sweet Potatoes and Green Saute

DAY 7:

Breakfast: Garlic and Ginger Beef

Lunch: Sweet and Sour Stir Fry

Snacks: Beef or Lamb Bone Broth

Dinner: Simple Chuck Roast

DAY 8:

Breakfast: Roasted Butternut and Red Pepper Soup

Lunch: Lo Mein

Snacks: Sweet Potato Stuffing

Dinner: Dairy Free Mac and Cheese

DAY 9:

Breakfast: Chicken and Turkey Broth

Lunch: Baked Potatoes and Fennel

Snacks: Basic Pork Bone Broth

Dinner: Sautéed Kale with Pasture Butter

DAY 10:

Breakfast: Chicken Bone Broth Lemon Loaf

Lunch: Simple Greens Soup

Snacks: Quinoa Pesto Salad

Dinner: Savory Turkey Rice

DAY 11:

Breakfast: Beef and Winter Vegetable Soup

Lunch: Super Skin Care Bone Broth

Snacks: Grain-free Sausage and Stuffing

Dinner: Dairy Free Scalloped Potatoes

DAY 12:

Breakfast: Energy Booster Bone Broth

Lunch: Nightshade-free Pizza

Snacks: Bone Broth and Celery Soup

Dinner: Simple Chuck Roast

DAY 13:

Breakfast: Breakfast Soup

Lunch: Tomato and Oregano Soup

Snacks: Greens and Sweet Potatoes Sauté

Dinner: Beef Stroganoff

DAY 14:

Breakfast: Energy Booster Bone Broth

Lunch: Bacon and Orzo Soup

Snacks: Bacon Mushroom Liver Pate

Dinner: Vietnamese Noodle Soup

DAY 15:

Breakfast: Strong Immunity System Bone Broth

Lunch: Savory Turkey Rice

Snacks: Matzoh Ball Soup

Dinner: Green Bean Casserole

DAY 16:

Breakfast: Basil and Carrot Soup

Lunch: Gut Healing Bone Broth

Snacks: Slow-Cooked Crispy Caramelized Pork Noodle Soup

Dinner: Garlic Chowder

DAY 17:

Breakfast: Strong Immunity System Bone Broth

Lunch: Cornbread with thyme and cranberries

Snacks: Butternut Squash Risotto

Dinner: Mexican Chicken Soup

DAY 18:

Breakfast: Gut Healing Bone Broth

Lunch: Sausage and Kale Bake

Snacks: Spinach and Arugula Salad

Dinner: Roasted Chicken with Orzo Soup

DAY 19:

Breakfast: Anti-Inflammation Bone Broth

Lunch: Beef Broth Tortellini

Snacks: Quinoa Flakes

Dinner: Lemongrass and Ginger Poached Halibut

DAY 20:

Breakfast: Duck, Chicken and/or Turkey Bone Broth Soup

Lunch: Butter Lettuce Wraps with Egg Salad

Snacks: Chicken Wings with Buffalo Sauce

Dinner: Paleo Cauliflower Soup

DAY 21:

Breakfast: Anti-Inflammation Bone Broth and Eggs

Lunch: Duck Mousse

Snacks: Spicy Tomato Salad

Dinner: Avocado Sandwich with sea salt and lemon juice

CHAPTER 3

BASIC BONE BROTHS

The basics are a very good place to start. Choose from any of these basic recipes to get started on your bone broth journey. You can then customize and create your own recipes to suit your personal tastes.

CLASSIC CHICKEN BONE BROTH

Makes 15 servings

Calories per cup: 86

Ingredients:

- 7 1/2 quarts filtered water
- 7 1/2 lb chicken feet, backs, and/or necks, raw
- 3 Tbsp apple cider vinegar
- 1 1/2 Tbsp sea salt
- 5 fresh thyme sprigs (optional)

Instructions:

1.
Place a large heavy-duty skillet over medium high flame and heat through. Cook the chicken parts in their own fat until

browned all over. Drain the oils thoroughly.

2.

Put the cooked chicken parts in a slow cooker, stockpot, or pressure cooker, then pour in the water. Stir in the vinegar and salt, then cover. Bring the mixture to a boil over high flame. Once boiling, reduce to a simmer and cook for up to 48 hours in the slow cooker, up to 24 hours in a stockpot over low flame, or up to 3 hours in a pressure cooker.

3.

Add more water, if necessary, and occasionally remove the film and fat that accumulated on the surface. Add the herbs, if using, right before the end of cooking time.

4.

Pour the broth through a mesh strainer and discard the bones and herbs, if using. Season to taste with salt, then let cool slightly and store in separate containers.

DUCK, CHICKEN AND/OR TURKEY BONE BROTH

Makes 15 servings

Calories per cup: 88

Ingredients:

- 7 1/2 lb duck, chicken, and/or turkey bones, raw
- 7 1/2 lb filtered water
- 3 Tbsp apple cider vinegar
- 1 1/2 Tbsp sea salt
- 6 fresh rosemary sprigs (optional)

Instructions:

1.

Place a large heavy-duty skillet over medium high flame and heat through. Cook the poultry parts in their own fat until browned all over. Drain the oils thoroughly.

2.

Put the cooked poultry parts in a slow cooker, stockpot, or pressure cooker, then pour in the water. Stir in the vinegar and salt, then cover.

3.

Bring the mixture to a boil over high flame. Once boiling, reduce to a simmer and cook for up to 48 hours in the slow cooker, up to 24 hours in a stockpot over low flame, or up to 3 hours in a pressure cooker.

4.

Add more water, if necessary, and occasionally remove the film and fat that accumulated on the surface. Add the herbs, if using, right before the end of cooking time.

5.

Pour the broth through a mesh strainer and discard the bones and herbs, if using. Season to taste with salt, then let cool slightly and store in separate containers.

BASIC PORK BONE BROTH

Makes 15 servings

Calories per cup: 90

Ingredients:

- 7 1/2 quarts filtered water
- 7 1/2 lb pork feet and/or bones, raw
- 3 Tbsp apple cider vinegar
- 1 1/2 Tbsp sea salt
- 2 Tbsp black peppercorns (optional)

Instructions:

1.

Place a large heavy-duty skillet over medium high flame and heat through. Cook the pork bones in their own fat until browned all over. Drain the oils thoroughly.

2.

Put the cooked pork bones in a slow cooker, stockpot, or pressure cooker, then pour in the water. Stir in the vinegar and salt, then cover.

3.

Bring the mixture to a boil over high flame. Once boiling, reduce to a simmer and cook for up to 48 hours in the slow cooker, up to 24 hours in a stockpot over low flame, or up to 3 hours in a pressure cooker.

4.

Add more water, if necessary, and occasionally remove the film and fat that accumulated on the surface. Add the peppercorn, if using, right before the end of cooking time.

5.

Pour the broth through a mesh strainer and discard the bones and peppercorns, if using. Season to taste with salt, then let cool slightly and store in separate containers.

CLASSIC BEEF BONE BROTH

Makes 15 servings

Calories per cup: 66

Ingredients:

- 7 1/2 quarts filtered water
- 7 1/2 lb beef marrow bones, raw
- 3 Tbsp apple cider vinegar
- 1 1/2 Tbsp sea salt
- 3 bay leaves (optional)

Instructions:

6.

Place a large heavy-duty skillet over medium high flame and heat through. Cook the beef bone parts in their own fat until browned all over. Drain the oils thoroughly.

7.

Put the cooked beef bones in a slow cooker, stockpot, or pressure cooker, then pour in the water. Stir in the vinegar and salt, then cover.

8.

Bring the mixture to a boil over high flame. Once boiling, reduce to a simmer and cook for up to 48 hours in the slow cooker, up to 24 hours in a stockpot over low flame, or up to 3 hours in a pressure cooker.

9.

Add more water, if necessary, and occasionally remove the film and fat that accumulated on the surface. Add the herbs, if using, right before the end of cooking time.

10.

Pour the broth through a mesh strainer and discard the bones and herbs, if using. Season to taste with salt, then let cool slightly and store in separate containers.

LAMB BONE BROTH

Makes 15 servings

Calories per cup: 88

Ingredients:

- 7 1/2 quarts filtered water
- 7 1/2 lb lamb marrow bones, raw
- 3 Tbsp apple cider vinegar
- 1 1/2 Tbsp sea salt
- 3 whole cloves or 6 fresh mint sprigs (optional)

Instructions:

1.

Place a large heavy-duty skillet over medium high flame and heat through. Cook the lamb bone parts in their own fat until browned all over. Drain the oils thoroughly.

2.

Put the cooked lamb bones in a slow cooker, stockpot, or pressure cooker, then pour in the water. Stir in the vinegar and salt, then cover.

3.

Bring the mixture to a boil over high flame. Once boiling, reduce to a simmer and cook for up to 48 hours in the slow cooker, up to 24 hours in a stockpot over low flame, or up to 3 hours in a pressure cooker.

4.

Add more water, if necessary, and occasionally remove the film and fat that accumulated on the surface. Add the herbs, if using, right before the end of cooking time.

5.

Pour the broth through a mesh strainer and discard the bones and herbs, if using. Season to taste with salt, then let cool slightly and store in separate containers.

FISH BONE BROTH

Makes 15 servings

Calories per cup: 40

Ingredients:

- 7 1/2 quarts filtered water
- 7 1/2 lb fish carcasses and heads, raw
- 3 Tbsp apple cider vinegar
- 1 1/2 Tbsp sea salt
- 6 fresh dill sprigs (optional)

Instructions:

1.

Place a large heavy-duty skillet over medium high flame and heat through. Add the fish bones and just enough water to cover them. Cover the skillet and simmer until steamed.

2.

Pour the cooked fish bones along with any remaining liquid from the skillet in a slow cooker, stockpot, or pressure cooker, then pour in the water. Stir in the vinegar and salt, then cover.

3.

Bring the mixture to a boil over high flame. Once boiling, reduce to a simmer and cook for up to 48 hours in the slow cooker, up to 24 hours in a stockpot over low flame, or up to 3 hours in a pressure cooker.

4.

Add more water, if necessary, and occasionally remove the film and fat that accumulated on the surface. Add the herbs, if using, right before the end of cooking time.

5.

Pour the broth through a mesh strainer and discard the bones and herbs, if using. Season to taste with salt, then let cool slightly and store in separate containers.

VENISON BONE BROTH

Makes 1 gallon or about 15 servings

Ingredients

- Approx. 5 lbs. of Venison Bones with some meat attached
- 3 tbsp. of Apple Cider Vinegar
- 4 tbsp. of Coconut Oil or Organic Animal Lard
- 1 Tbsp of crushed Juniper Berries (this is optional)
- Additions for at the last hour of cooking if desired
- 1 tbsp. of Sea Salt
- 1 tbsp. of Black Peppercorns
- 2 tbsp. of Rosemary
- 1 tbsp. of Thyme
- 5 Bay Leaves
- 1 medium sized Organic Onion chopped
- 2 large Organic Carrots Chopped
- 2 large Organic Parsnips Chopped
- 2 medium sized Organic Celery Sticks sliced
- A good handful of fresh Organic Parsley

Instructions

1. Place the bones in a large heavy bottomed stainless stock pot and cover them with cold water. Place them over a medium heat and bring to the boil, then simmer them for 20 minutes.

2. Drain the water from them and place the bones on a roasting tray. If you wish to, you can cut them up using a bone saw or hack-saw, this will allow you to fit more bones into a smaller pot.

3. Use the coconut oil to oil the bones and then roast them in an oven at 400F (180C) until they are well browned

4. Place the bones in a heavy bottomed stock pot with enough pure fresh water to completely cover them and then bring the water to a steady boil, add the juniper berries and reduce the heat to a very low simmer, so the water steams a little, but does nor roll around.

5. Ideally, the broth should simmer for at least 12 hours, but 24 or more is ok. Occasionally skim off any froth that develops on the surface.

6. During the last 2 hours, you can add the remaining ingredients if you feel you must, our preference is to not add anything at this stage, just strain the bone broth through a cheesecloth lined colander or sieve to remove all the solids into a food safe container

7. Use some of the broth straight away, if you wish to add the extra ingredients at this stage would be a good time and any remaining should be placed in a shallow container which is in turn placed into a larger ice filled container to cool as quickly as possible.

8. Once cooled place the bone broth into a refrigerator for about 6 to 8 hours during which time any fat will come to the surface where it can be removed and used elsewhere. Place any broth you cannot use within a few days in the freezer to keep for longer

HOMEMADE FRENCH BREAD
GLUTEN FREE

This recipe for a healthy gluten free French Bread is created to compliment your bone broth, it is relatively easy to make and any extra will freeze well, so you can always have some available to enjoy with your bone broth

Ingredients

- 2 cups of Homemade or Organic Rice Flour
- 1 cup of Homemade or Organic Potato Flour
- 1 ½ tsp of Rock or Sea Salt
- 1 tbsp. of Konjac Powder (A seaweed extract that is available from most health food shops or online)
- 2 tbsp. of Raw Honey, Maple Syrup or Organic Raw Sugar
- 1 ½ cups of slightly warm water
- 2 tbsp. of Instant Organic Yeast
- 1 tbsp. of Organic Animal lard or Pure Unsalted Butter, melted
- 3 large Free Range Organic Egg Whites, beaten
- 1 tsp of Apple Cider Vinegar

Instructions

1. Place the rice flour, potato flour and konjac powder in a bowl and whisk it to aerate and fully combine (this can be done in the bowl of your electric mixer)

2. Place the warm water and honey in a small bowl and sprinkle in the yeast and allow it to begin working

3. Blend the yeast/honey mixture into the flours either by hand or using the dough hook on an electric mixer

4. Add the butter, egg whites and vinegar and beat the mixture on high for 3 minutes

5. Oil your baking sheet with animal lard, coconut oil of butter and then lightly dust it with cornmeal

6. Place the dough on the baking sheet using a spoon and shape into French loaves leaving enough space between for them to double in size

7. Make every 2 inches (5cm) a diagonal slash in the top of each loaf

8. Cover the loaves with a slightly damp cloth and leave them in a warm area to double in size

9. Bake the loaves in a preheated oven @ 400F (200C) for 30 to 35 minutes. When the bread is cooked remove them from the oven and allow to cool on wire racks.

CHAPTER 4

HEALTH-BOOSTING BONE BROTHS

Want something a little bit more than the basics? Master these recipes to gain specific health and beauty benefits!

SUPER SKIN CARE BONE BROTH (COLLAGEN- AND LYCOPENE-RICH)

Makes 5 servings

Calories per cup: 88

Ingredients:

- 1 1/2 lb. pig feet
- 1 1/2 lb. chicken feet
- 2 1/2 quarts filtered water
- 1/2 lb. tomatoes, chopped
- 1 Tbsp apple cider vinegar
- 1/2 Tbsp sea salt
- 1/2 hot red pepper (optional)

Instructions:

1.

Place a large heavy-duty skillet over medium high flame and heat through. Add the pig feet and chicken feet and just enough water to cover them. Cover the skillet and simmer until steamed.

2.

Place the cooked bones along with any remaining liquid from the skillet into a pressure cooker or slow cooker, then pour in the water. Stir in the vinegar and salt, then cover.

3.

Cook for 2 hours in the pressure cooker or for 24 hours in the slow cooker. Add more water, if necessary, and occasionally remove the film and fat that accumulated on the surface. Add the tomatoes and red pepper, if using, near the end of cooking time.

4.

Pour the broth through a mesh strainer and discard the bones and pepper, if using. Season to taste with salt, then let cool slightly and store in separate containers.

STRONG IMMUNITY SYSTEM BONE BROTH (ANTIOXIDANT AND ANTIBACTERIAL)

Makes 5 servings

Calories per cup: 90

Ingredients:

- 2 1/2 lb. chicken bones, raw
- 1 Tbsp apple cider vinegar
- 2 1/2 quarts filtered water
- 2 oz. dried maitake mushrooms
- 2 oz. dried shiitake mushrooms
- 1 garlic bulb, halved
- 1/2 Tbsp sea salt
- 3 fresh oregano sprigs

Instructions:

1.
Soak the mushrooms in water until reconstituted. Drain and set aside.

2.
Place a large heavy-duty skillet over medium high flame and heat through. Cook the chicken parts in their own fat until browned all over. Drain the oils thoroughly.

3.

Place the cooked bones into a pressure cooker or slow cooker, then pour in water. Stir in the vinegar and salt, then cover.

4.

Cook for 2 hours in the pressure cooker or for 24 hours in the slow cooker. Add more water, if necessary, and occasionally remove the film and fat that accumulated on the surface.

5.

After de-pressurizing the pressure cooker, or two hours before the end of cooking time in the slow cooker, stir in the garlic, mushrooms, and oregano.

6.

Pour the broth through a mesh strainer and discard the solids. Season to taste with salt, then let cool slightly and store in separate containers.

ENERGY BOOSTER BONE BROTH

Makes 5 servings

Calories per cup: 88

Ingredients:

- 2 1/2 quarts filtered water
- 2 1/2 lb.

Instructions:

- 2 1/2 lb. chicken, beef or salmon bones, raw
- 3 inches fresh lemongrass, crushed
- 1/2 bunch asparagus, chopped
- 1 Tbsp apple cider vinegar
- 1/2 Tbsp sea salt

Instructions:

1.

Place a large heavy-duty skillet over medium high flame and heat through. Cook the chicken or beef bones in their own fat until browned all over. Drain the oils thoroughly. If using salmon bones, steam in water until cooked through.

2.

Place the cooked bones into a pressure cooker or slow cooker, then pour in the water. Stir in the vinegar and salt, then cover.

3.

Cook for 2 hours in the pressure cooker or for 24 hours in the slow cooker. Add more water, if necessary, and occasionally remove the film and fat that accumulated on the surface.

4.

After de-pressurizing the pressure cooker, or two hours before the end of cooking time in the slow cooker, stir in the asparagus and lemongrass.

5.

Pour the broth through a mesh strainer and discard the solids. Season to taste with salt, then let cool slightly and store in separate containers.

ANTI-INFLAMMATION BONE BROTH

Makes 5 servings

Calories per cup: 91

Ingredients:

- 2 1/2 quarts filtered water
- 2 1/2 l lamb or beef marrow bones, raw
- 1 small sweet potato, quartered
- 3 inches fresh ginger root, sliced
- 2 fresh turmeric roots, sliced
- 1 Tbsp apple cider vinegar
- 1/2 Tbsp sea salt

Instructions:

1.
Place a large heavy-duty skillet over medium high flame and heat through. Cook the beef or lamb bones in their own fat until browned all over. Drain the oils thoroughly.

2.
Place the cooked bones into a pressure cooker or slow cooker, then pour in the water. Stir in the vinegar and salt, then cover.

3.
Cook for 2 hours in the pressure cooker or for 24 hours in the slow cooker. Add more water, if necessary, and

occasionally remove the film and fat that accumulated on the surface.

4.

After de-pressurizing the pressure cooker, or two hours before the end of cooking time in the slow cooker, stir in the ginger, turmeric, and sweet potato.

5.

Pour the broth through a mesh strainer and discard the solids. Season to taste with salt, then let cool slightly and store in separate containers.

GUT HEALING BONE BROTH (BILE AND DIGESTIVE JUICE STIMULANT, MILD LAXATIVE, BLOOD GLUCOSE STABILIZER AND INTESTINE SOOTHER)

Makes 5 servings

Calories per cup: 91

Ingredients:

- 2 1/2 quarts filtered water
- 2 1/2 lb. chicken, beef or salmon bones, raw
- 2 small beet roots, cubed
- Greens from beet roots
- 1 medium zucchini, sliced
- 1 Tbsp apple cider vinegar
- 1/2 Tbsp sea salt

Instructions:

1. Place a large heavy-duty skillet over medium high flame and heat through. Cook the chicken or beef bones in their own fat until browned all over. Drain the oils thoroughly. If using salmon bones, steam in water until cooked through.

2. Place the cooked bones into a pressure cooker or slow cooker, then pour in the water. Stir in the vinegar and salt,

then cover.

3. Cook for 2 hours in the pressure cooker or for 24 hours in the slow cooker. Add more water, if necessary, and occasionally remove the film and fat that accumulated on the surface.

4. After de-pressurizing the pressure cooker, or two hours before the end of cooking time in the slow cooker, stir in the beets and zucchini.

5. Pour the broth through a mesh strainer and discard the solids. Season to taste with salt, then let cool slightly and store in separate containers.

CHAPTER 5

BONE BROTH MAIN DISHES

Who knew soups can become great main dishes? Cook your favorite vegetables and meats in bone broth and you will feel instantly satisfied! Those who aspire to lose weight will want to enjoy the soups alone, but if you want, you can add a delicious dinner roll on the side.

SPRING VEGETABLE SOUP

Makes 4 servings

Calories per cup: 150

Ingredients:

- 1/4 Tbsp olive oil
- 1 large red skinned potato, scrubbed and chopped
- 1/2 cup chopped leek, white and green parts
- 1/2 lb. asparagus, trimmed and chopped
- 1/2 cup frozen peas, thawed
- 1 quart fish bone broth
- 1/2 tsp sea salt
- 1/4 tsp freshly ground black pepper
- 4 Tbsp light sour cream (optional)

Instructions:

1.

Place a soup pot over medium high flame and heat the olive oil.

2.

Stir in the leek and cook until tender, then stir in the potatoes and broth. Season with salt and pepper to taste and bring to a boil.

3.

Once boiling, reduce to medium low flame and stir in the asparagus and peas. Simmer for 5 minutes or until asparagus is tender.

4.

Ladle into four soup bowls, then top with sour cream and serve right away.

ROASTED BUTTERNUT AND RED PEPPER SOUP

Makes 4 servings

Calories per cup: 119

Ingredients:

- 1 Tbsp olive oil
- 1 small butternut squash
- 4 medium bell peppers
- 2 1/2 cups beef or lamb bone broth
- 1/4 tsp freshly ground black pepper
- 1/2 tsp sea salt
- 1/4 tsp smoked paprika

Instructions:

1.
Set the oven to 375 degrees F. Line a baking sheet with parchment paper and coat with a bit of olive oil.

2.
Slice the butternut squash in half and discard the seeds.

3.
Arrange the halved squash and bell peppers on the prepared baking sheet and drizzle a bit of olive oil over them. Season with salt and pepper.

4.

Bake for 45 minutes, then remove the bell peppers and bake the squash for an additional 5 to 10 minutes, or until very tender.

5.

Carefully remove the skins off the bell peppers and scoop the squash flesh out of the shell.

6.

Chop up the bell peppers and squash and place in a bowl. Pour in the hot broth and add the smoked paprika. Serve right away.

BEEFY VEGETABLE SOUP

Makes 4 servings

Calories per cup: 199

Ingredients:

- 1/2 Tbsp vegetable oil
- 3/4 lb. organic minced sirloin
- 1 carrot, diced
- 1 parsnip, diced
- 1 celery rib, diced
- 1/2 cup diced yellow onion
- 1/2-quart beef bone broth
- 1 cup water
- 1 cup chopped tomatoes, juices reserved
- 1 Tbsp chopped fresh flat leaf parsley
- 1/4 tsp dried thyme
- 1/2 bay leaf
- 1/2 tsp sea salt
- 1/4 tsp freshly ground black pepper

Instructions:

1.
Place a soup pot over medium flame and heat the olive oil. Sauté the celery, parsnips, and carrots until tender. Move to

the side of the pot.

2.

Stir in the beef and sauté until cooked through, then combine with the diced vegetables.

3.

Add the broth, tomatoes with the juices, water, bay leaf, thyme, parsley, salt and pepper. Increase to high flame and bring to a boil.

4.

Once boiling, reduce to a simmer and cook for about 15 minutes.

5.

Remove the bay leaf, then serve.

SIMPLE GREENS SOUP

Makes 4 servings

Calories per cup: 99

Ingredients:

- 1 cup chopped fresh kale
- 1 cup chopped fresh collards or chard
- 3 1/2 cups beef or pork bone broth
- 1/2 Tbsp grass-fed butter
- 1/4 cup fresh flat leaf parsley
- 2 Tbsp freshly squeezed lemon juice

Instructions:

1.
Chop the kale and collards or chard into the thinnest possible strips. Set aside.

2.
Pour the broth into a soup pot and place over medium flame. Bring to a simmer, then stir in the greens. Cover and let simmer for 3 minutes, or until the greens are wilted.

3.
Turn off the heat, then stir in the butter, parsley and lemon juice. Serve right away.

CREAM OF CAULIFLOWER SOUP

Makes 3 servings

Calories per cup: 109

Ingredients:

- 1/2 cauliflower head, chopped into florets
- 1 cup chicken bone broth
- 2 Tbsp grass-fed butter
- Freshly ground black pepper, to taste

Instructions:

1.
Combine the chopped cauliflower florets and chicken broth in a soup pot and place over high flame.

2.
Cover and let boil. Once boiling, reduce to a simmer and cook for 10 minutes, or until the cauliflower is extremely tender, but not mushy.

3.
Turn off the heat, uncover, and let cool slightly.

Once cooled, transfer the florets into a food processor or blender and add the butter and some of the broth. Blend until creamy, then stir back into the pot and serve. Reheat before serving, if desired.

CURRIED LENTIL SOUP WITH COCONUT MILK

Like a great bone broth, this lentil soup takes time to prepare and cook, but it is equally like a great bone broth which it is made with well worth the effort both in its flavor and health promoting properties.

Serves 6 to 8

Ingredients

Half a gallon (2lit) of Chicken Bone Broth

- 1 ½ cups of Yellow Lentils
- ½ a cup of Red Lentils
- 2 tsp of Live Yogurt, Fresh Lemon Juice or Apple Cider Vinegar.
- 1 tsp of Coriander Seed
- 1 tsp of Coriander Seed
- 1 tsp of Cumin Seed
- 1 tsp of Fenugreek Seed
- 6 whole Cardamom Pods
- 2tbsp of Organic Animal Lard or Ghee
- 1 medium Organic White Onion finely sliced
- ½ inch piece of Organic Ginger finely minced
- 1 tsp of Curry Powder
- 1/4 of a tsp of Cayenne Pepper
- 1 tsp of Oyster or Fish Sauce

- 1 cup of Sundried Organic Raisins
- 2 cups of fresh or full Coconut Milk

To Serve

- 1 cup of live Organic Yogurt
- ½ a cup of Fresh Parsley (Cilantro)
- A little Fresh Lime Juice

Instructions

1. Place the yellow and red lentils in a bowl with the 2 tsp of Live Yogurt, Fresh Lemon Juice or Apple Cider Vinegar and then fill with hot water to cover them by 2 inches, and set aside for 10 to 12 hours. Once they have been soaked the lentils must be rinsed thoroughly and then drained.

2. Heat a heavy skillet over a moderate heat and heat until reasonably hot then place the coriander, fenugreek cumin and cardamom seeds inside to roast for about 2 minutes stirring constantly to get them evenly toasted. Remove them from your skillet and crush them in a mortar and pestle of if preferred in a spice grinder (coffee grinder works well)

3. Place the lard or Ghee into a heavy bottomed saucepan and heat it to a moderate heat, sauté the onions and ginger until fragrant about 3 minutes and then stir in the toasted spices, curry powder and cayenne pepper, cotinine to sauté for several minutes longer

4. Place the chicken bone broth into the saucepan with the rinsed and drained lentils and the oyster sauce. Once the soup is boiling, it is time to reduce the heat to a low simmer and continue cooking until the lentils are tender approximately 45 minutes.

5. Use a stick blender or a bench blender to puree the soup and then stir in the coconut milk and the raisins. Simmer the soup for a further ten minutes before serving with the yogurt, cilantro and the fresh Lime.

FRENCH ONION SOUP

French Onion soup is an old time favorite with many people and most do not realise just how nutrient rich it is if made with the best available

For 4 to 6 servings

Ingredients

- 2 liters or ½ a gallon of Beef Bone Broth
- 8 to 10 large Organic White or Brown Onions
- 4 or 5 cloves of Organic Garlic (or more if preferred)
- 1Tbsp of Organic Animal Lard or Coconut Oil
- Freshly ground Black Pepper and Sea Salt to Taste

- A Bouquet Garni made using 2 large stalks of Parsley, 2 sprigs of Thyme and 2 Bay Leaves tied together
- Some fresh Wholesome Croutons
- Some Grated Tasty Cheese
- A small amount of finely chopped Parsley or other Herb or a Garnish

Instructions

1. Slice the onions finely and place them and the lard in a heavy bottomed stock pot and sauté them for a few minutes or until tender.

2. Add the broth and simmer the soup for about 20 minutes

3. Taste the soup and adjust the seasoning, adding salt and or black pepper, then remove the banquet garni.

4. Lightly toast the croutons and place the soup into serving bowls with the croutons on top of the soup, sprinkle a generous amount of cheese on top and a sprinkling of chopped parsley.

5. Place under an overhead grill to melt and slightly brown the cheese just before serving.

CHICKEN NOODLE SOUP

As already discussed earlier chicken soup is one of the older time honoured and proven home remedies that have been used for many years and is still popular today, its benefits are immense if made with wholesome natural ingredients including chicken bone broth.

Serves 4 to 6 people

Ingredients

- 2 liters or ½ a gallon of Chicken Bone Broth
- 1 Organic Carrot thinly sliced
- 1 Organic Onion thinly sliced
- 1 large stick of Organic Celery with the leaves included
- 3 to 4 cloves of fresh Organic Garlic crushed
- A small piece of green Ginger crushed
- A small piece of Turmeric crushed (optional)
- ½ a cup of assorted Organic Green Leafy Vegetables
- Any other Fresh Organic Vegetable you may have
- Some diced fresh organic Chicken Pieces or cooked shredded Chicken
- Fresh Homemade Pasta Noodles Or Organic Egg Noodles
- Freshly Ground or Cracked Black Pepper and Sea Salt to taste

Instructions

1. Wash all the vegetables and slice them thinly or grate them as required

2. Place the broth in a large heavy bottomed saucepan and bring it to a slow simmer, add all the vegetables except the green leafy items.

3. If the chicken is raw add it now or if already cooked add with the noodles later

4. Simmer the soup until everything is tender, this will take about 20 minutes in a saucepan or 3 minutes in a pressure cooker.

5. Add the noodles, green leafy vegetables and chicken if already cooked and simmer for a few minutes.

6. When the noodles are tender, before serving, taste and adjust the seasoning if necessary and then serve.

PORTABLE BONE BROTH, HOMEMADE BOUILLON

Our forefathers used portable bone broth in years past, as a valuable staple which was often used by many travellers in many lands, long before the modern equivalent of "A cup of Instant Noodles" became popular and many modern cooks reached for instant stock cubes or canned powdered bouillon to make their soups stews and sauces. These modern manufactured alternatives to real bone broth can contain many different types of nasty chemical ingredients including processed fats MSG and refined salt. With many of these commercially produced broths there is no real bone or meat content many used soy or other bases. There is no real substitute for a well-made, organic broth, both for health and flavor.

Makes about gallon

Ingredients

- 10 lbs. of Free, Organic, Meaty Bones Chicken, Beef, Lamb, Pork etc. or a mixture if desired
- 2 tablespoons of Black Peppercorns
- 2 Bay or Laurel Leaves
- 2 teaspoons of Sea or Rock Salt (unrefined)
- 2 tablespoons of Organic Free Range Gelatine if desired this can be left out if you are using bones that contain a lot of natural gelatine such as feet knuckles and sinew

Instructions

1. Preheat your oven to about 450 F

2. Place all the bones on a tray or oven dishes and roast them for at least 45 minutes

3. Place all of the bones in a large heavy bottomed stock pot with the peppercorns and bay leaves. Fill the pot with enough fresh drinking water to completely cover the bones by several inches and bring the water to a steady boil on a medium to high heat. Reduce the amount of heat until the bones are simmering and allow it to keep simmering for between 12 and 24 hours

4. Alternatively, you can use a pressure cooker and reduce the cooking time to 3 to 4 hours.

5. When you determine that the broth is ready, turn off the heat, and allow it to cool to a temperature that is safe to handle and pass it through a strainer or cheesecloth lined colander to remove any particles.

6. Cool the broth to cool to room temperature and place it in a food grade air tight container to be refrigerated for between 8 to 12 hours, but no longer than 24 hours. During this time all the fat will rise to the surface, where it can be collected and saved to be used in other applications, (please note that this fat is extremely nutritious and should not be wasted)

7. Place the broth in a wide mouthed saucepan and simmer it, taste it and add salt accordingly, continue simmering until it reduces to about a cup or becomes very thick. Depending on the size of your saucepan and the depth of broth this should take about 45 minutes or it can be reduced in the oven in shallow baking trays on a low heat setting.

8. Often when making these we add a little homemade tomato paste for added flavor and nutrients, but this is entirely optional.

9. Whisk the gelatine into the hot broth and then pour the broth into food safe containers at about 3 to 4 inches deep and allow this to cool and then refrigerate for about 8 to 12 hours.

10. Cut the broth/bouillon into about 1 inch cubes and place them gently on a dry cotton cloth placed in a cool place or in the refrigerator for another 12 to 24 hours.

11. These cubes will remain usable if kept in an airtight food safe container at room temperature of 8 to 12 months.

12. When required simply place a cube in a cup of hot water to dissolve as a drink or use it to flavor soups sauces and stews.

AUTHENTIC OYSTER SAUCE

Oyster sauce is so similar to bone broth and equally if not easier to make at home as long as you can get some fresh sea caught Oysters.

There are only 2 ingredients

- Fresh Oysters and enough clean unpolluted Sea Water to cover them, or if unavailable use pure fresh drinking water with sea salt added, About 1 tablespoon to each litre of water.

-

Instructions

1. Wash the outside of the oyster shells and place them in a large stainless steel or enameled saucepan and cover them with plenty of sea water.

2. Bring the water to a steady fast simmer and cook until the water is reduced to about half about then strain the liquid and return it to the saucepan.

3. Further reduce the liquid until it becomes thick and sauce-like.

4. This sauce will keep refrigerated for about 12 months.

BASIC BROWN SAUCE

When you have your own supply of bone broth, you can very easily make all your own extremely tasty and healthy sauces to accompany any meal. As arguably the best French Chef ever, the legendary Augusta Escoffier was known for saying such things as "indeed, stock and broth are everything in cooking. Without it. Nothing good can be done"

Ingredients

- 1 cup of Homemade Bone Broth
- 1 cup of a good drinking Dry Red Wine
- 3 tbsp. of Organic unsalted Butter
- 3 tbsp. of Organic Flour
- 3 medium sized Spring Onions or ½ of a Red Onion
- A fresh Bouquet Garni made using 3 Basil leaves, a Sprig of Thyme and a Bay Leaf tied in a bundle or a ¼ teaspoon of dried Thyme
- Sea Salt and Fresh Cracked Black Pepper to taste

Instructions

1. Sauté the onions in the butter until golden brown, soft and tender
2. Add the flour stirring until it has absorbed all the butter and cooked through, allow it to brown but do not burn

3. Add the red wine, stock and the bouquet garni stirring constantly to produce a thick smooth sauce, Simmer for about 3 minutes, taste and season if necessary with the cracked black pepper and sea salt.

4. This sauce can be enriched by adding some homemade tomato paste or oyster sauce

5. Demi-glace is traditionally made as a base for other sauces as well as being a rich sauce in its own right. To make this extra rich sauce add equal parts of brown sauce and bone broth and reduce this back down to half again or to the consistency you like for the dish you are serving.

RED GRAVY

Gravy's have for years had a bad rep as being unhealthy, but this depends on the ingredients you decide to use making them. These types of gravies are healthy because they are made from the finest wholesome ingredients with no processed additives.

Ingredients

- 3 cupsful of Homemade Bone Broth
- 3 cupsful of Homemade or Organic Tomato Sauce
- ½ of a cup of Homemade or Organic Tomato Paste
- ½ a cup of Organic Animal Lard
- 15 cloves of Organic Garlic sliced into quarters
- 1 large Organic Onion Diced
- 1 tbsp. of freshly minced Sweet Basil or 1 tsp of dried
- 1 tbsp. of freshly minced Thyme or 1 tsp of dried
- A Bouquet Garni made with 1 Bay Leaf, a sprig of Rosemary and a piece of fresh lemongrass
- 11/2 tsp of ground Cayenne Pepper
- 1 tsp of freshly cracked Black Pepper
- 2 tsp of Sea Salt

Instruction

1. Place the lard in a heavy bottomed saucepan and heat it to a moderate and sauté the garlic until

golden.

2. Remove the garlic and sauté the onions until they soften and start to turn brown being careful not to burn them

3. Add the tomato paste and stir while cooking, so the onions become coated

4. Add the rest of the ingredients and allow the mixture to simmer for about 45 minutes.

5. Taste the gravy and add the seasoning if necessary, Remove the bouquet garni before serving.

STIR-FRIED VEGETABLES

We have all for many years known that Chinese style stir-fried vegetables are one of the healthiest ways of eating, this is largely because of the quick cooking time helps to retain many of the nutrients. Recent studies have revealed that by using a broth as a cooking liquid instead of oil or fat many of the heat sensitive nutrients and even many enzymes can also be retained. This is because the cooking temperature is further reduced and the food is semi streamed but still retains its crunchiness plus you get the health benefits of the broth, which also helps to enhance the flavor.

4 serving

Ingredients

These ingredients are suggestions and any fresh local vegetables should be used in preference.

- ½ of a cup of Organic Broccoli sliced or Broccoli Shoots sliced
- ½ a cup of Organic Cauliflower sliced into flowerets
- 1 small Organic Onion sliced
- 1 small Organic Capsicum sliced
- 3 stalks or Organic Celery Sliced
- ¼ of a cup of Organic mushrooms sliced
- ¼ of a cup of Organic Baby Corn
- ½ a cup of Organic Cabbage
- 1 tbsp. of Organic Green Ginger finely shredded
- 3 cloves of Fresh Organic Ginger finely chopped

- ½ of a tbsp. of Fresh Turmeric very finely diced or 1 tsp of Organic Turmeric powder (Optional)
- 1 cup of your preferred free range Organic sliced meat or Seafood's
- 1 cup of Bone Broth
- 1 tbsp. of Homemade Oyster Sauce (Optional)
- 1 tbsp. of Cold Pressed Coconut Oil

Instructions

1. If you are using fresh meat it is a good idea to sauté it first and then remove it from the wok while the vegetables cook. Most seafood's are best added at the last minute of cooking time to retain their flavor and tenderness.

2. Place your wok, a large fry pan or saucepan on a medium heat and add about half a cup of bone broth. When this has reached boiling point add a tablespoon of coconut oil or olive oil.

3. Add the finely shredded turmeric, ginger and garlic and stir to coat then add the carrots, allow this to cook for several minutes and add all the rest of the vegetables.

4. Add the balance to the broth Plus more if needed and the oyster sauce,

5. Season with fresh cracked black pepper and sea salt of you did not use the oyster sauce.

6. Serve as soon as ready to avoid spoiling by over cooking

PRESSURE COOKED CHICKEN

Naturally raised chickens take much longer to grow to a good size for eating than factory farmed birds that are given growth stimulants and hormones along with a cocktail of horrendous chemicals to grow large in a few weeks. For this reason, they are seldom as tenders as the fancy store bought chicken breasts most people are familiar with. But they are much more flavor full and contain many beneficial nutrients.

This recipe uses organic free ranged and fed chicken as well as broth made from the same free range organic chickens. Be sure when you finish your meal to keep the bones to make some more delicious bone broth. Any poultry can be used for this recipe with each different type of bird providing its own unique flavor.

For 4 to 6 people

Ingredients

1. 2 & ½ cups of Chicken Bone Broth
2. 1 whole naturally fed free range Chicken
3. 3 Organic Sweet potatoes cut into portion sizes
4. 3 to 6 portions of Organic Pumpkin
5. 1 Head of Organic Broccoli
6. 1 Head of Organic Cauliflower
7. 3 to 6 whole small organic Carrots
8. 1 small Organic Onion
9. 1 small Organic Orange
10. 4 Cloves of Organic Garlic

11. 1 small Piece of Organic Ginger

12. 1 small piece of Organic Turmeric

13. 1 stalk of Organic Lemon Grass

14. 4 whole Star Anise pods

15. 1 large sprig of Thyme

16. 3 Bay leaves

17. ¼ of a tsp of whole Peppercorns

18. 1 tsp of Sea Salt

19. 2 tbsp. of Flour

Instructions

1. Wash all the vegetables and crush the ginger, turmeric and Garlic with a mallet or heavy knife

2. Rinse the chicken and rub the inside with sea salt then stuff it with the orange, onion, ginger, garlic, turmeric, lemongrass and thyme.

3. Place the chicken broth in the bottom of the pressure cooker with the bay leaves, star anise and peppercorns then place in the stand or internal plate to keep the chicken out of the liquid.

4. Place the chicken inside the pressure cooker and attach the lid, following the manufacturer's user instruction for safety.

5. Turn on the heat and allow the cooker to reach the operating temperature required in the instructions.

6. Allow the chicken to cook for 5 to 7 minutes and turn off the heat. The pressure ill drop and you will be

able to open the lid.

7. Place the sweet potatoes, carrots and pumpkin inside and reset the lid.

8. Turn on the heat and allow the cooker to operate for 3 minutes more then turn off the heat again allowing the pressure to drop so you can once again open the cooker

9. Add the broccoli and cauliflower and any other vegetable you may want to eat and replace the lid. Turn on the heat and cook for about 2 minutes and then turn off the heat again. Allow the cooker to cool down so you can safely open the lid and remove the vegetables and chicken. When removing the chicken tilt it, so all the liquid inside (and there I likely to be a considerable amount) will drain back into the cooker.

10. Using a whisk blend the remaining juices inside the cooker with the flour to create a rich sauce. Turn on the heat again without the lid, stir the sauce constantly for a few minutes to ensure it has cooked then taste it and adjust the seasoning if necessary. You may find you wish to add some homemade oyster sauces tomato paste or extra bone broth.

11. The sauce can be strained if you wish we usually just place it in the blender for a few minutes and enjoy the benefits of all the ingredients.

12. Do not forget to keep the bones for your next batch of healthy bone broth, as soon as they cool down they can be frozen or hung out to dry.

13. By making a simple salad while this healthy and tasty meal cooks you can enjoy a full meal in less

than 30 minutes, a meal that will satisfy even the most discerning person (or fussy eaters).

HEARTY BEEF STEW

This beef stew recipe is ideal for using budget priced cuts of meat, often the lesser priced or budget cuts of meat that actually have the same or even more nutritional values as the more expensive cuts. There is no reason why if you desire a substitute for the beef any other type of livestock can be used instead. Just for your health's sake ensure you only eat livestock that has been raised in the proper way such as free range pasture and naturally or organically fed with access to sunshine and fresh air and not from commercial feedlots where the conditions of overcrowding and commercial unnatural feeds make the meat hazardous to your health.

If you wish to cook this stew quickly, then I suggest you use a pressure cooker to reduce the cooking time to about 30 minutes. Some of the best results can come from using a pressure cooker or crock-pot.

Serves 4 to 6 people

Ingredients

- 500g of Organic Beef diced into cubes
- 2 cups of Bone Broth (preferably Beef but any Homemade Bone Broth works)
- 2 Organic Onions diced
- 2 Organic Carrots cut into rings
- 2 Organic Beets diced
- 2 Organic Parsnips, Turnips, Swedes or a mixture diced
- 1 cup of Organic Pumpkin diced

- ½ a cup of Organic Button Mushrooms
- 4 cloves of Organic Garlic (or more) diced
- 1 piece of Organic Ginger (1/2in) crushed
- 2 tbsp. of Organic or Homemade Tomato Paste
- 2 tbsp. of Organic or Homemade Oyster Sauce
- ½ a tsp of Black Peppercorns
- 2 Bay Leaves
- 2 to 4 Star Anise Pods
- 1 tsp of Sea Salt
- 2 tbsp. of Organic Lard or Coconut oil

Instructions

1. Place the lard in a heavy bottomed saucepan and brown the beef on all sides
2. Add the onions, garlic and ginger and sauté until softened then add the bone broth, tomato paste, oyster sauce, bay leaves, star anise and peppercorns.
3. Simmer the stew for about 2 hours and check the meat for tenderness (some of the cheaper cuts will take longer to cook)
4. When the beef is tender add the rest of the ingredients including the vegetables and simmer for another 30 minutes.

To cook using a Pressure Cooker or Crock-Pot,

For the best results, first, sear or brown off the beef on all sides.

5. If using the Pressure cooker, place the beef with the bone broth, ginger, bay leaves star anise salt inside and cook for 15 minutes, then turn off the heat allowing the cooker to cool so you can open it to add the rest of the ingredients including the vegetables

6. Close the lid and turn on the heat cooking for a further 10 minutes, then turn off and allow it to cool

7. Check the meat for tenderness and taste and adjust the seasoning, if the meat is not tender cook for a further 5 minutes and check again

To cook this Stew in a Slow Cooker or Crock-Pot

8. Place all the ingredients in your crock-pot and cook or about 12 hours, stirring occasionally.

CHAPTER 6

BONE BROTH REMEDIES

On days when you are feeling under the weather, sipping some bone broth on top of following your doctor's prescriptions will definitely help!

THE ANTI-ALLERGY REMEDY

Makes 2 servings

Calories per cup: 88

Ingredients:

• 1 cup chicken bone broth (or **Strong Immunity System Bone Broth**)

• 3 Tbsp apple cider vinegar

• 1 cup organic Nettle Tea

Instructions:

1.
Prepare the nettle tea based on the manufacturer's instructions.

2.

Pour the broth into a small pot and place over low flame. Heat through, then stir in the tea and apple cider vinegar.

3.
Pour the mixture into a mug and serve right away.

THE COUGH CURE

Makes 2 servings

Calories per cup: 92

Ingredients:

• 1 cup chicken bone broth (or **Strong Immunity System Bone Broth**)

• 4 Tbsp raw honey

• 4 drops therapeutic grade eucalyptus or peppermint essential oils (optional

• 1 1/2 cups filtered water

• 1/2 cup fresh thyme leaves

Instructions:

1.
Pour the filtered water into a small pot and add the thyme leaves. Brew, uncovered, over medium low flame for 20 minutes, or until only about half of the water is left.

2.
Meanwhile, pour the broth in a larger pot and heat through over medium flame. Turn off the heat.

3.
Strain the thyme leaves from the tea and pour the tea into the broth. Stir in the essential oil, if using, and honey until the honey is completely dissolved.

4.

Pour into a mug and serve right away.

THE LOSE WEIGHT REMEDY

Makes 2 servings

Calories per cup: 88

Ingredients:

- 2 cups beef or lamb bone broth (or **Super Skin Care Bone Broth**)
- 3 Tbsp apple cider vinegar
- 1/3 cup freshly squeezed lemon juice

Instructions:

1.
Pour the broth into a small pot and place over low flame. Heat through, then turn off the heat.

2.
Stir in the apple cider vinegar and lemon juice. Pour into a mug and serve right away.

THE COMFORT FOOD / ANTI-FEVER REMEDY

Makes 2 to 3 servings

Calories per cup: 123

Ingredients:

- 2 cloves garlic, peeled
- 1 onion, chopped
- 1 small, free range whole chicken or turkey
- 1 gallon water
- Cayenne pepper, to taste
- 1 Tbsp. peppercorns
- 2 Tbsp. apple cider vinegar
- 4 stalks celery, chopped
- 4 oz. shitake mushrooms
- 2 carrots, chopped

Instructions:

Put all of the ingredients in a slow cooker or crockpot, and then cover and boil for 24 hours.

Skim off any impurities that will come to the surface during the first 2 to 5 hours of cooking, and then strain through a bowl. Discard meat or any other food particles, as well.

Store in mason or glass jars, and use in a matter of 5 days. You can also freeze the broth and use it for at least a month!

THE DETOXIFYING BROTH / ANTI FREE RADICALS

Makes 2 to 3 servings

Calories per cup: 24

Ingredients:

- 1 celery rib, chopped
- 1 medium yellow onion, chopped
- 2 Tbsp. butter
- 1 carrot, chopped
- 1 green apple, cored, peeled and chopped
- 1 butternut squash, de-seeded, peeled and chopped
- 1 gluten-free cooking broth
- 1 cup bone broth
- 3 cups chicken or vegetable broth
- 1 cup evaporated milk
- A pinch of nutmeg, cayenne, salt, pepper or cinnamon

Instructions:

Melt butter in a large pot or saucepan over medium heat before adding garlic and onion. Add apples and sprinkle nutmeg on top.

Stir for around two minutes then add the vegetable or chicken broth, squash and cumin. Bring the mixture to a boil and simmer after reducing heat.

Pour contents in a blender or food processor together with evaporated milk and puree the mixture until smooth.

Bring the mixture back to the saucepan and simmer for around 5 minutes in low heat. Season with salt and pepper, to taste.

Serve and enjoy!

CHAPTER 7

WHERE TO FIND BONES FOR YOUR BONE BROTH

A problem that some bone broth practitioners face is that they have no idea where to find good bones for your bone broth. Well, this might also be something that you're asking yourself. Maybe, you're wondering if you should just ask the butcher, or the people at the grocery to save you some, right? It could be so confusing that you might feel like you won't be able to make the diet work for you, but hey, don't fret: there are a lot of solutions to your problems.

There are actually a number of ways for you to get the right kinds of bones for your bone broth. If you live in New York, there's this store called *Brodo* at the East Village which is a bone-broth only takeout counter, so that's a good thing. However, if you do not live near the mentioned area, you can just go to the market or the grocery—your local ones will do—and buy bone-in meat. You can cook the meat however way you want, and boil the bones to get bone broth. After all, it would definitely be a hassle to travel to New York solely for the purpose of getting "good bones" when you can actually get them in your area.

FEET AND KNUCKLES

Some people who make bone broth also suggest that you get feet and knuckle bones as they provide not just bones and broth, but also gelatine that contains collagen which is also good for your gut, especially if they're grass-fed. These parts are also surprisingly so juicy, which means there's a lot that you can make out of them!

WHOLE FOODS AND MORE

Fresh Markets and *Whole Foods* are also said to have a good selection of bones, with Whole Foods having "bag of bones" being sold at the freezer section. They'd cost you just around $3, or even less, and you'd already get a big bag of them. You may also find frozen chicken carcasses at Whole Foods, taken from pastured or free-range chicken—those could give you amazing broth, too, and there might be lots of meat attached there, too, so you can use those to cook the recipe you have in mind. Aside from *Whole Foods,* Kroger also has a bone section in the freezer area, so you might want to check that out, too.

If there's no Whole Foods or any of those popular groceries in your area, you can try asking your own local butcher if he has any spare bones left, and chances are, he would have some. Asian and Spanish grocery stores usually have this policy, so it's best that you go and ask the butcher.

GO ONLINE

If all else fails, you can check out *Coombe Farm Organic* or *Eat Wild,* websites that sell marrow bones and organic stock. They also have cuts that are deemed hard to find so you might be able to make amazing purchases here, especially if you are in the UK. They even have lists of butchers who save those bones so you'd be able to ask them for help.

See, there are various ways for you to find those bones—all you have to do is look!

CHAPTER 8

HOW TO ENHANCE THE USE OF BONE BROTH

Yes, it's a given: cooking bone broth can be tricky, but it's definitely doable. When it comes to cooking bone broth, here's what you have to keep in mind:

1. Get a large stock pot, and place the bones there. Use water to cover the bones with.

2. Get some apple cider vinegar, about two tablespoons, and add it to the water. Do this before cooking. If apple cider vinegar is not available, you can just use wine, instead. This way, you can get more nutrients from the bones.

3. Get some filtered water, and then pour it into the pot. Make sure there is plenty of room that will be left for boiling.

4. Heat the pot slowly, and start boiling. Reduce heat, and let it simmer for at least 6 hours—make sure to be wary of scum and remove it as it makes its way to the surface.

5. Remember to cook slow and long, and take note that bones of chicken cook way for at least 6 to 48 hours, and beef bones take longer—at least 12 to 72 hours. Cooking in the right time frame will definitely help you get all the minerals and nutrients you need.

You will then notice that after cooking, a layer of fat would be floating on top. Don't be scared of this, for it is responsible of protecting the broth—and helping keep nutrients in check.

BOOST YOUR BROTH WITH...

You can provide more acidity for the broth—and also give it more flavor, and enhance nutrients found in it by making use of broth boosters, such as the following:

Whole Nutmeg + Cinnamon Sticks + Cloves + Star Anise + Fresh Ginger

Thyme + Sage + Rosemary

Peppercorns + Lemon + Dried Fennel

Lemon and Green Tea Bags (make sure to add tea only during the last 5 minutes of cooking!)

Jalapenos + Cayenne Pepper (Jalapenos should be added during the last 20 minutes of cooking)

Garlic + Scallions (Garlic should be added during the last 30 minutes of cooking)

Fennel Root + Star Anise

Dill and Lemon

TAKING CARE OF THE STOCK

You can also turn the broth into stock, which you can use for most recipes—a few of which you'll find in the following chapter. Making stock out of the broth is good because if you are not fond of slurping broth alone, it would be good to know that you can just add it to recipes that you'll be making. It not only gives more flavor to your recipes, it will also help you get all the nutrients you need in a much easier fashion.

What you can do is place some bones in a stockpot or crockpot, and then cover the bones with cold water. Set the temperature to low, and then add 2 Tbsp. of apple cider vinegar so that you will be able to start getting minerals from the bones. Roast beef bones for at least 25 to 30 minutes prior to boiling, if you want, to get more flavor from your stock.

Beef and other tough bones take at least 6 minutes to cook, if you're going to make stock out of them, and chicken cooks for around 4 hours. If you want to season the stock, wait until cooking time is about to be over—at least 10 minutes before the end—and then go and add spices and fresh herbs. Spice powders could be added in the last hour, and you can just add vegetables according to their size.

Stews and gravies would work well with nutmeg, while fenugreek powder and turmeric would work great for soups.

For stews and soups, you can also use *bouquet garni,* which is a mixture of bay leaves, rosemary, and thyme. You can place them in a pouch, or have them tied together, and then add fresh peppercorns to make it spicier. Meanwhile, you can use *mirepoix,* or a mixture of onions, celery, and dried carrots. These provide great taste for your recipes, and are even used in French cuisine.

CHAPTER 9

OTHER AMAZING BENEFITS OF BONE BROTH

Aside from the remedies it could bring, there are a lot more amazing things that bone broth can do, and these are the following.

EASY DETOXIFICATION

One of the best things that bone broth can do for you is that it makes way for easy detoxification.

You see, bone broth contains glycine, a mineral that helps produce stomach acid, regulating the digestive process, and making sure that you'd have enough energy, even if you're fasting. When your body consumes glycine, muscle is not broken down by the body, so you will have good stature—minus the fats, of course.

Your body actually has its own detoxification system, namely the liver, and with the help of Glycine, you can be sure that the liver would be able to make enough sugar fuel. The sugar fuel can be used in the absence of glucose.

The body also uses glycine for glutathione synthesis, which means you'll be able to get the most important antioxidants around. These antioxidants, aside from fighting free radicals that destroy cells in the body, and making sure that you get healthy, supple skin, also aids in the production of endogenous antioxidants. When these are around, oxidative stress can easily be combated—and you'll get to absorb Vitamin C more.

Excess methionine in the body can also be cleared out. While the body needs it—as it is an amino acid—too much of it can cause blood levels to rise, which isn't good. This also helps you realize that eating every part of the animal is good, because it means that you get a good balance of minerals that your body actually needs.

PROPER DIGESTION

Other diets—and the food you eat—may make digestion hard, and that's not exactly what you want to experience in life.

Again, bone broth has glycine which produces stomach juices that the body needs. Stomach acid deficiency can make your body weaker, and can make your immune system more susceptible to diseases, mostly because it allows half-digested food to stay in the stomach. Thus, it results in indigestion, and acid is forced up towards the esophagus, which can be quite painful.

If you may recall, the liver is also in charge of producing bile —which is a good mineral used for the digestion of fat in the small intestine, and can also help you normalize your blood levels. Mostly, this is good for people who are just trying out the Paleo Diet.

Bone broth is also a natural remedy for leaky gut, mostly because it produces glutamine, an amino acid that makes sure your gut works well alongside your body. This way, negative autoimmune reactions can be prevented. This also improves the condition of your intestinal wall, so further damage can easily be prevented.

JOINT PROTECTION

Bone broth is great when it comes to protecting your joints.

Bone broth has glucosamine that allows your joints to be pain-free, and healthy. Not only that, bone broth also has chondroitin sulfate that helps prevent osteoporosis—which means your bones would be healthy and strong enough to support you all along.

Speaking of osteoporosis, minerals calcium, magnesium, and phosphorous—these are all seeped in the broth, and when you get them in your body, you'll definitely be able to protect your bones much better.

AMAZING IMMUNE SYSTEM SUPPORT

Bone broth works like superfoods. Why? Well, simply because it has this high concentration of minerals, and in fact, according to Mark Sisson, the author of *The Primal Blueprint,* bone marrow naturally strengthens the immune system—and when you get the broth from it, you'll be able to absorb these nutrients even better, keeping you safe from most ailments and diseases. In fact, it even works like chicken soup—in the sense that it easily makes you feel better.

IT HELPS YOU SLEEP BETTER

And, bone broth also helps you sleep better—all thanks, to glycine.

In short, this has mostly everything that you need to help you cruise well in life—and that's why you've got to add it to your diet as soon as you can!

Printed in Great Britain
by Amazon

48196562R00064